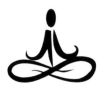

# KEEP CALM
## AND BREATHE

10 Deep Breathing Techniques
to Bring Awareness, Relieve Stress,
Reduce Anxiety, and Change Your Life
Forever!

By: Julie Schoen

# CONTENTS

# FOREWORD

Last fall I watched my grandfather's health begin to decline. At ninety years old, he had beaten cancer, struggled with seizures, received a pacemaker, and had cataract surgery on both eyes. My grandfather has always been a tough guy, serving in the U.S. Army during World War II. I could see his toughness each time he re-covered from a health issue; he seemed stronger and bolder than before. That is why it came as such a shock when I received a call from my mom telling me that my grandfather, my tough guy, had taken a turn for the worse. When I asked about what was going on, what was damaging his health and threatening his life, I was surprised by the answer: panic attacks.

My grandfather, an engineer always wanting to be in control of everything and understand the innermost workings of every gadget that came into his home, was struggling with the thought of death. Death was not something he could understand. He couldn't break it apart, like the radios he used to work on in the war, and see how it worked. He couldn't control it. He had no idea when he would die, how it would happen, what it would feel like – and the fear of that was causing him to experience debilitating panic attacks. He couldn't sleep, having to call my parents to his home in the middle of the night to sit with him, assuring him that he was going to be okay. My grandmother was becoming exhausted by his constant demands.

Doctors began to prescribe medication, but every pill he took seemed to create a new problem: dizziness, depression, thoughts of suicide. At ninety, it seemed like his body just couldn't handle the powerful drugs that many people swear by. My family became desperate.

As a yoga instructor, I understand the power of breathing; I teach it in every class, reminding my students to feel their breath, to stay focused on their breath, to move with their breath. I wanted to give my grandfather a lesson in deep breathing, hoping that the connection between the breath and the body and mind would help him recover from his attacks and reclaim his life.

We started slowly, working on feeling the breath enter and exit the body. I asked him to listen to his body, to get in tune by recognizing how it changes with every inhalation, every exhalation. We started taking deeper breaths, filling the lungs more fully and exhaling completely. I told him to imagine all of his fears and anxiety leaving his body with every exhalation and to feel his body relax when he did so. On the inhalations, he began to visualize positive thoughts entering his body. He began to feel the power of love from his family every time he inhaled.

I opened my eyes to look at my grandfather during one of our breathing sessions and, to my surprise, I saw a smile on his face, a smile that hadn't been seen in the months since he began experiencing panic attacks. I asked him how he was feeling and he simply replied, "I feel so light." We continued the deep breathing exercises and within minutes he was dozing off to sleep, finally relaxed and freed from the fears that had been holding him captive for months.

This is just one of the stories I have watched unfold as someone, sometimes for the first time, learns how to breathe.

The potential power you have with every breath you take is astonishing. You have the ability to change your life, literally in every way possible, just by taking the time to practice deep breathing exercises each day. Deep breathing is simple, it takes only a few minutes, and anyone can do it. There is no one on this planet that cannot benefit from learning how to breathe effectively.

There is an old yogic saying that says **you are only given a certain amount of breaths in your lifetime, so by slowing your breath down, you slow death down.** My hope is that this book will improve your life and inspire you to appreciate every breath you take.

And remember, Keep Calm and Breathe!

With Love,

*Julie*

# APPRECIATING YOUR PRANA

It is estimated that each day the average person takes upwards of 21,000 breaths. With the very first moment of life, our breath is with us constantly, providing us with a life sustaining force. **The way we breathe influences all processes of the body**, from the obvious functioning of the lungs to the reactions of our nervous system, our mind and body are directly linked to our breath. Within minutes of losing oxygen, the brain and the body's vital organs will shut down and, if breathing does not start again, within seconds life can end. Breathing is so important that the body regulates it for us, making it possible to sleep and complete day-to-day tasks without having to think about each inhale and exhale.

**But what would happen if we became conscious of our breathing patterns?**

The ancient practice of yoga, which was developed over 5,000 years ago in India, asks its followers to do just that. Pranayama, a Sanskrit word that, when broken down, literally means "controlling or directing life energy", teaches practitioners to not only observe their breath, but also how to direct and control it throughout the body. The result of this conscious breathing is the ability cope with stress and anxiety as it arises and, most importantly, a means for living in the present moment, experiencing the joys of life instead of just simply allowing them to pass us by.

Prana, or "life force", is the key to being peaceful, healthy, and content. The equation is simple; the more prana you have, the better you feel, physically, mentally, emotionally, and spiritually. And just how do you lure this "life force" into your body? The answer is simply by breathing.

## Apana Vs. Prana

According to yoga masters, prana is brought into the body with each inhale, but (and this is an important but) only if there is room for it. Yogis believe that bad habits, negative thoughts, stress, anxiety, and unhealthy bodies create something known as "apana", which is basically a Sanskrit word for "rubbish". If your body is filled with apana then there can be no room for the prana you are trying to inhale in. Unfortunately, you can't just set your apana on the side of the road and wait for it to be picked up. Getting rid of apana takes work. One must be able to control their breathing in order to consciously exhale the body's garbage out.

## Conscious Breathing Leads To Improved Health

When you begin to take notice of your breath, at first just by observing it, you will notice that the quality of your breathing is directly linked to the way your body functions, including how your mind thinks. **There is a positive cycle that is created when you learn** to increase the quality of your breathing: **the more quality of breath leads to more quality of mind leads to more quality of life which leads back to quality of breath.** According to the yoga legend BKS Iyengar, "Evenness of breathing leads to healthy nerves and so to evenness of mind and temper." Iyengar goes on to say that practicing specific breathing techniques on a regular basis "will change the mental outlook of the practitioner and reduce considerably the craving of his senses for worldly pleasures", such as smoking and drinking.

In order to appreciate your prana you must learn the difference between consciously observing it, which includes skillfully directing it through your body, and forcing the breath to do what you want. The reason many of us feel fear and anxiety is precisely because our bodies take control of the breath, wanting to aggressively maintain an impossible state. When this happens, the body tenses, the breath is stopped, and negative thoughts and feelings set in.

## Free Yourself of Friction

The goal of practicing specific breathing techniques is to learn to adapt to change and to free the breath. Whether we like it or not, our environment is in a constant state of flux. Therefore, if we cannot move with it, if we resist change and strive for stasis, there will be friction. This friction, unfortunately, is something that many people have grown far too accustomed with. Today, over nineteen million people suffer from anxiety. On any given day, thirty to fifty percent of the world will not be able to sleep because of insomnia. And, according to recent estimates, about 121 million people worldwide suffer from some form of depression.

If you are placed on a treadmill you have two choices. You can either run with it, adjusting to the speed and the incline as it changes, or you can refuse to move, which results in a painful fall with cuts and burns from the friction of the moving belt. Learning to appreciate your breath, to observe it as it changes and to direct it through your body, is the equivalent of deciding to run on the treadmill. It doesn't mean that life won't get hard, but when it does, you will be far better equipped to accept the changes, to modify your body's reaction, and to return to a new state of ease.

# THE BASICS OF BREATH

Putting deep breathing exercises to use may seem easy and why shouldn't it? Breathing is something we have been practicing since before we were born. But the kind of breathing that must be cultivated in order to successfully practice true Pranayama is something that is brand new to the majority of us. At its base, breathing is nothing more than something that keeps us alive. **At the pinnacle of breath, however, is a healing force that improves the functioning of the body, calms the nervous system, provides limitless energy and can even help people cure illnesses and fight life-threatening issues such as obesity and high blood pressure.**

So before you begin practicing the deep breathing techniques that follow, there are a few basics you should be familiar with so that you can take your breathing from simply life sustaining to something that is a powerful healer. These basic tips are to help you begin to shift your mindset and to start viewing your breath as a vital tool you have been given to improve your health and your overall well-being.

### Time and Place

Setting a specific time and place for practicing different deep breathing techniques helps you to create intention, making it easier for you to focus. Although many of the deep breathing techniques discussed can be used "in the heat of the moment", when you begin to feel stressed, anxious, or lethargic, it is best to not think of breathing exercises as useful on a purely need basis.

**Practicing conscious breathing on a consistent basis at the same time and place each day will prevent you from feeling desperate throughout your day.** Regular breathing work can be thought of as a daily multivitamin or preventative medicine, the more you practice, the less you will feel like you need it, which is the exact reason why you should practice more!

According to BKS Iyengar's classic yoga guide, *Light On Yoga*, **"the best time for practice is in the early morning (preferably before sunrise) and after sunset."** In the morning, it is thought that your body can gain power and energy from the sun as it rises, making it an ideal time for practicing breathing exercises and preparing your mental attitude and outlook for the day.

Ideally, you should find a place to do deep breathing that is quiet and free from distractions. Similar, if not exact, to meditation, you need a place where you can be completely comfortable, both mind and body, in order to keep you from feeling restless.

## Posture

Speaking of being comfortable and free from distractions, how you sit when you are practicing deep breathing is incredibly important. If you pick a seat that is uncomfortable, you will not be able to focus solely on your breath, which means that you will not receive the benefits and, most likely, you will give up on a daily Pranayama practice.

Here are some suggested postures that are ideal for deep breath work. Most importantly, however, is that you are comfortable, your spine is straight and erect (even if you are lying down), and that there is no effort to maintain that posture for several minutes. Keep in mind that a position that may start as comfortable can quickly prove to be uncomfortable as time progresses.

## Suggested Postures For Deep Breathing:

- Sitting on the floor with your legs crossed. If you have a blanket on hand, fold it a few times and sit on the very edge of it to help keep your lower back free from unnecessary strain.
- Sitting on top of your heels with your knees bent and legs together, tops of the feet flat on the floor. Some people find this pose very comfortable, while others feel discomfort in their knees and ankles, especially if they stay in the posture for an extended period of time.
- Sitting on the edge of a chair or stool with your feet flat on the ground, shins perpendicular to the floor and thighs parallel to the floor. Be sure to sit up tall without overarching your back or slumping your shoulders.

- Lying flat on the floor with your entire spine and shoulders coming in contact with the ground. There are lots of ways to find comfort in this pose, such as bending the knees to relieve pressure from the low back and placing a pillow under your head. There are, however, certain deep breathing exercises that cannot be practiced in this posture, especially the ones with forceful breathing, such as skull breathing.

### Training Your Senses

One of the essential keys to being successful when practicing deep breathing exercises is learning to tune into your senses, learning to turn off your mind to outside distractions and focus it instead on your body and breath. Similar principles that are taught in meditation can be very useful to learning how to consciously breathe.

Your mind must have one point of focus, which, for the most part in Pranayama, is the breath. **There are several aspects of the breath which can become your focal point, the sound, the feel, the direction of movement, and, of course, the count.** When focusing on the sound, you will notice the distinct difference between your inhale and exhale and will begin to recognize changes as you try a variety of the exercises discussed later. The feel of the breath also changes with the inhalation and exhalation as well as with the type of deep breathing being practiced. Most likely, you will feel the breath move through the nose and cool the throat on the inhalation. On the exhale you will feel the breath leaving the body, feeling the lungs empty from bottom to top. By consciously directing the breath through the body and bringing it to the attention of your mind, you are developing a crucial skill in learning how to effectively breathe.

Finally, you can train your senses to tune into the breath count, which, for many people beginning to practice conscious breathing exercises, is the easiest. You can simply count the breath using nothing more than just your mind. Or you can use many of the tools people have come up with to deepen the focus, such as using a strand of beads to keep track of the number of breaths.

Traditionally, people practicing Pranayama use their hand to keep track of their breaths. It is ideal to take at least twelve deep breaths each time you sit down to practice deep breathing. Using your thumb, you can use the twelve different parts of your hand and focus your mind on moving your thumb to count each breath. (See the picture below for the traditional pattern of twelve.)

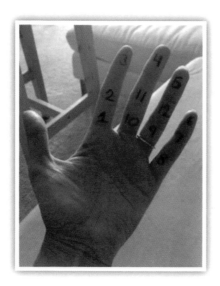

## Focus The Mind Using The "Internal Gaze"

Another cue to be taken from meditation is practicing the "internal gaze". It is amazing how often we move our eyes every minute, even when sleeping. By stilling the eyes, with the eyelids closed, we are actually giving the senses and the brain a much-needed break. To practice internal gazing, close your eyes and focus them on one point of your body, such as the tip of your nose, the spot between your eyebrows, or the navel. Direct your eyes to this part, keeping the gaze still and steady. This practice is actually much more difficult than it sounds, but it is incredibly helpful for keeping the mind focused so that you can breathe consciously without interruptions.

Finally, be sure to be paying attention to your body while you're breathing. It is important to never suppress the body's natural urges when practicing deep breathing exercises. If your body tells you that it really needs a breath, give it one! Conscious breathing is meant to soothe the body so if your body is sending out signals that it is feeling stressed, listen to it and make the necessary changes.

# THE BREATH BODY CONNECTION

The way we breathe is intrinsically connected to our body. Our bodies react to changes that we make to our breath and our breath changes as a reaction to our bodies. For example, when a woman is in labor she is reminded time and time again to breathe, as slow and steady as possible. One of the main reasons she receives this instruction is because by relaxing her breath, her body will also relax, making it more capable of delivering a baby because her body can adapt to the variety of demands.

Imagine a marathon runner in the 24th mile of their 26-mile race. Their body is exhausted and their breath has become labored. There are two choices they can make, give into their exhausted body and, therefore, have their breath react to the body or they can begin to consciously breathe, directing the breath to their exhausted muscles and, therefore, having their body react to their breath. In the first scenario, the body will collapse in exhaustion.

However in the second scenario, where the power of the breath is recognized, **the runner is able to keep going because their body is positively reacting to their controlled breath**.

There are three different ways in which the connection between body and breath can manifest, **collapsing, propping, and yielding**. Collapsing of the body occurs when we give in to the forces of gravity and the result is a tired and lethargic body, lacking in self-confidence, marked by a shallow breathing pattern.

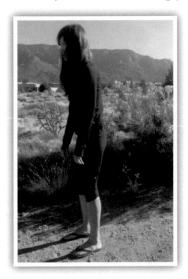

Propping of the body is the normal reaction people have when they realize that they are collapsing. A propped body is being forced to stand erect, pushing the ground away with great force, tight legs, and locked knees. In order to keep your body in this position, a lot of willpower and energy is required. The result of propping your body is an overactive nervous system, which makes you anxious and nervous and your breath labored and forced.

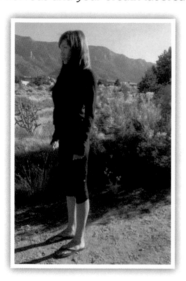

**The ideal in-between state is yielding – learning to give in to gravity while simultaneously pushing against it**. This state reflects the dynamic flux of the breath, which allows energy and oxygen (prana) to move freely throughout the body, not being controlled like it is when the body is propped and not completely unconscious as it is when the body collapses. **Learning to allow your body to yield creates a state of balance that will free you of anxiousness and anger while helping your body to heal and energize itself**. When you yield, you consciously direct the breath through the body, sending it where it is most needed.

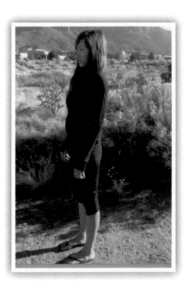

Yielding is a fine balancing act of push and pull; learning to breathe while yielding is no different. You must be conscious, but not forceful. You direct the breath through the body, but you do not strain to do so. Learning how to breathe effectively takes time and, like anything, the more you do it the easier it becomes. As long as you are conscious of your breath you will begin to notice its relationship to your body. Armed with that knowledge, you will know how to change your breath in order to change your body and mind.

*Always remember that the quality of your breath expresses your inner feelings, what is going on in your mind and body. Changing your breath can change your life.*

# 10 DEEP BREATHING TECHNIQUES TO TRANSFORM YOUR LIFE

The following deep breathing exercises are each unique in what they are meant to accomplish, **some are used to energize the body, while others are used to soothe the mind and calm the nervous system**. Regardless of which breathing technique you choose to practice, all of them share in their ability to make you conscious of your breathing. Some of the techniques are much more challenging than others and will take time to master. Others may seem very basic, but should not be overlooked as they can provide soothing effects and a deeper awareness of your breath and how it affects your body.

Unless specified, all breathing exercises should be performed using the nostrils only.

*As a note, if you are pregnant or have medical concerns it is best advised to not retain the breath. You should also refrain from practicing breath retention if you are not able to practice comfortably and relaxed.*

### Conscious Breathing – Feeling The Power Of Your Breath

In order to begin to breathe consciously, you must be able to feel how the breath affects your body. In this exercise you should choose a posture that allows your body to freely move. For example, you can stand with your feet hip-width apart and knees dramatically bent. Allow your body to fall forward over your legs, draping the head, neck and arms. You can mimic this same posture sitting in a chair.

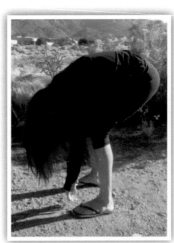

Turn your senses inward and begin to consciously notice your breath as it enters and leaves your body. Simply observe how the breath begins to move your body, expanding with inhales and condensing with exhales. Allow your body to move freely with your breath, joining body and breath together in one fluid motion. Let your body be light and relaxed. Feel the lightness of your bones and muscles, almost as if you are floating in water.

Your body will only begin to truly be moved by the breath once you make a conscious effort to stop controlling and to simply allow yourself to be moved. Let your body participate with the breath and the feel the freedom that comes from no longer forcing a state of control. If you are finding it difficult to relax into the process of conscious breathing, exhale deeply through the mouth several times, relaxing your jaw and mouth and relieving built-up tension.

**Breathing With The Body – Allow The Breath to Soothe You**

This exercise is great to use if you sense your breath becoming shallow or restricted. The movement that comes from the marriage of breath with body frees the breath and relaxes the body and mind. You can perform this technique anytime, anywhere without drawing attention because the movement is incredibly subtle. You will notice that even the slightest movement when practiced with an awareness of breath will immediately soothe your mind.

Sitting in a comfortable posture, place your hands palms up on your thighs. Allow the fingers to stretch open, but do not force them to become completely extended. Then let the fingers relax, gently curling into your palm. With intention, begin to create a rhythm of curling and uncurling your fingers. Bring awareness to your breath and notice the relationship between each breath, the inhalation and exhalation, and the movement of your hands.

You can go deeper into this exercise by bringing your awareness to your chest and spine, noticing the same subtle link between the movement of your body and your inhalation and exhalation.

### Guided Breath – Heal Your Body From Stress and Tension

This exercise allows you to tap into your inner body, taking time to see which areas are straining or holding tension. Over time you will notice that your body reacts to stress and anxiety by tightening muscles and "gripping". For example, some people will realize that every time they get angry or stressed, their jaw tightens. For others, their shoulder may tense or the muscles around their hips and lower spine might get tight. Practicing guided breath will help you see your body's reaction to negative emotions and will therefore help you ease the tension and stress you are experiencing.

In a comfortable seated posture, turn your focus inward, quieting the mind and practicing "internal gazing", directing your closed eyes to one point on your body. Starting from the crown of your head and working your way down the body, do an inventory of your muscles and joints. Which ones are tight? Which ones are gripping? Which ones are sore or tense?

As you discover tightness and tension in your body, begin to direct the breath to those areas. Visualize the breath moving through your body, penetrating and healing each cell. As the breath reaches that area, feel the tension melt away. Once you feel completely at ease, remain in the posture for several more breaths, quietly absorbing the healing power of each and every breath.

### Learn To Yield – Receive a Relaxed State of Mind

*"Any surface of the body that makes contact with the ground must yield to the earth. Actively yielding to the earth creates a rebounding force away from the earth, elongating the body upward into space. Whenever the relationship of yielding to the earth is lost, breathing is restricted."* – Donna Farhi

As discussed previously, **learning to yield is a fine balancing act that, when mastered, frees your breath to move smoothly and easily throughout the body.** When you experience ease of breath, maybe for the first time in your life, you will notice the dramatic effects it has on your body and mind. **Completing tasks becomes easier. Your mind becomes alert. Stress and anxiety are freed from the body and positive thoughts are allowed to enter.** When the breath is allowed to do what it was meant to do, which is more than just keeping us alive, obstacles that have troubled you in the past will be much easier to overcome.

It is best to practice this yielding exercise in a standing posture. First feel the differences between collapsing, propping, and yielding. When you collapse, it feels as if you have no bones or muscles. You allow gravity to pull you down completely and your body begins to sink into the earth. Notice how your breath and mind react to this action.

Next feel your body propped, actively pushing the earth away, tensing the muscles of the legs, buttocks, and abdomen. Lift your chest up and squeeze your shoulder blades together. Again, notice how your breath and mind react to this action.

Now you are ready to feel the difference as you yield. As you exhale, feel your legs pressing into the earth. As you inhale, feel the energy from the earth rebound back into your body, lifting you upwards. As you practice feeding your energy down and receiving energy up, be sure to remove tension from your toes, feet, ankles, knees, hips, and buttocks. Pay attention to your breath as you practice and feel the difference between yielding and the two opposites, collapsing and propping. Notice the relaxed yet energized state of your mind.

### Soft Belly Breathing – Overcoming Fear and Anxiety

The core of your body is the source of all movement and energy. If your belly is constantly hard and tight with a feeling of being "held in" you are restricting the movement of both your energy and breath, creating very real, very negative consequences for your internal organs and your nervous system.

This practice is most easily done lying down flat on your back with one hand placed on your belly. Feel yourself breathe and notice if you are allowing your breath to enter your core. If you are, your belly will feel soft and mobile. If you are restricting your breath, it will feel tight. Donna Farhi, author of *The Breathing Book*, likens a hard belly to "a crashed car in the middle of an intersection – nothing can flow through it until the obstruction is removed".

Focus your mind on simply observing your breath, using your hand on your belly as a reminder to keep your core soft and mobile. Throughout your day, you may notice that certain circumstances will create tightness in your belly, use this exercise so that you can be aware of it happening and then simply use your exhale as a release, returning your belly to a soft and mobile center for energy to flow through.

### Full Chest Breathing – Unleash Your Body's Full Potential

Oftentimes people breathe very shallowly without even being aware of it. Shallow breathing has negative effects for several reasons. The first being very obvious – with your body receiving less oxygen it will not be able to function at its full capacity. Another reason that shallow breathing can be detrimental is because it creates a negative cycle. If you do not exhale fully you retain stress, anxiety, and fear. If you do not inhale fully you do not give your body the opportunity to fill itself with positive prana (life force) and energy. As your body fills with the negative emotions that you are not completely exhaling, it is filling up with what can be considered garbage (apana) and not leaving any room for positive change when an inhale is taken. This negative cycle is why it takes time, and a regular breathing practice, to fully feel the effects of the breath moving freely throughout the body.

**Full chest breathing helps you move from shallow breathing to full breathing, allowing you to more effectively rid the body of negativity and fill it with positive energy.** As you settle into your breathing practice, begin to consciously expand the chest and abdomen on the inhalation and consciously contract the abdomen on an exhalation.

As you inhale, feel the chest fill before you feel the abdomen fill. Do the opposite on the exhalation, emptying the abdomen before emptying the upper lobes of the lungs in the chest. On an inhalation feel the diaphragm moving downwards in order to allow your lungs to fill with breath. On an exhalation feel the front of the belly move towards the spine as the diaphragm moves up, helping to completely empty your lungs from bottom to top.

### Simple Cleansing Breaths – Creating Space for Positivity

It has been mentioned that in order to truly feel the amazing effects the breath can have your body, you must first cleanse the body of any rubbish (apana), which is things like fear, anxiety, nervousness, doubt, and low self-esteem. Negativity leaves the body through exhalations, so by emphasizing the exhalation you are more effectively able to cleanse the body, making room for the good energy you want.

In a comfortable posture, begin to observe your natural breath. If you can, notice which is naturally longer, the inhalation or exhalation? About how many counts is each of your natural inhalations? How many counts are your exhalations? Which is naturally easier, the inhalation or exhalation? Once you have become aware of your natural breathing pattern, you can begin the exercise of simple cleansing breaths, which consists of making the exhalation twice as long as the inhalation. Try starting with a count of four on your inhales and a count of eight on your exhales. You can modify the counts as needed, just ensure that you are never forcing the breath, rather you are simply guiding it.

### Alternate Nostril Breathing – Refresh Your Body and Mind

The goal of practicing this deep breathing exercise is to purify and balance the nerves of your body. Just as an obstruction in a water pipe can cut off your supply completely, obstructions in the nerves can have damaging effects to your body's ability to function regularly. Alternate nostril breathing supplies your blood with a boost of oxygen, leaving you feeling refreshed and calmed after practicing.

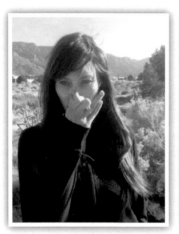 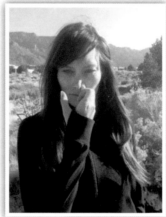

In a comfortable posture, bring your right hand to your nose with the index and middle finger bent towards the palm, fingers relaxed. The ring finger and pinky finger extend straight and towards the thumb. This hand position should feel relaxed and never forced.

Use your ring finger and pinky finger to close the opening of the left nostril; exhale completely through the opening of the right nostril. Then inhale slowly and deeply through the right nostril, filling the lungs completely. After a full inhalation, use the thumb to cover the right nostril and exhale through the left. Empty the lungs completely. Then take a full inhale through the left side, keeping the right side closed with your thumb. Once you have filled your lungs completely, close the left side with your ring and pinky finger and exhale fully on the right side.

This is one cycle of alternate nostril breathing. You can practice this technique for several minutes. Be sure to complete a full cycle before stopping, beginning and ending with an exhalation in the right nostril.

### Reclined Deep Breathing – A Specialized Technique with Super Benefits

This particular deep breathing exercise will do wonders for relieving fatigue and lowering blood pressure. The key for reaping the benefits of this technique is an emphasis on how the breathing is done. Also known as *ujjayi* in the yoga world, this type of breathing allows you to better guide the breath throughout the body because of a narrower passageway you create by slightly closing the vocal cords at the base of the throat. If you think of your breath like a hose, the wider the opening the less control you have of where the water goes. Of course then the opposite is also true, the smaller the opening the more control you have.

To understand this breathing technique, imagine your hand is a mirror or a window on a cold day. Hold your hand up to your face and exhale as if you wanted to the fog surface. Notice the audible "hmmm" sound that is produced when you do so. Now start to fog the surface again, but close your mouth halfway through the exhalation, maintaining the same position of your throat and the same (only slightly quieter) sound. Practice this a few times. Once you have mastered the exhalation, use the same technique on the inhalation, slightly closing the back of the throat and creating a soft but audible "sssss".

Lying down, continue to practice this type of breathing, inhaling and exhaling through the nose with the mouth closed. Notice the increased sense of control you have with this type of breathing. Focus the mind on the sound of the breath and feel your body reenergize.

## Skull Breathing – Reinvigorate Your Body, Mind, and Life

This advanced technique does not exactly qualify as a deep breathing exercise. In fact, it is quite the opposite, asking you to forcibly exhale at a rapid pace. **The effects of this type of breathing pattern, unlike many of the deep breathing exercises that soothe and calm the body, are an invigoration of the total body and a sense of exhilaration**. It helps to clear any fogginess that may be lingering in the mind and allows you to move forth in your day with clarity of mind and the energy to accomplish all of your tasks. Skull breathing is also very effective for cleansing air passages that may be blocked by mucus, such as sinus problems, or tension.

To practice skull breathing find a comfortable seated posture. Do not begin until your mind is focused and you have become aware of your breath. When you are ready to begin, take a slow inhalation through the nose and then forcibly exhale the air out through the nose, making an audible sound. As you exhale, the belly strongly pulls in towards your spine, helping you to expel more air from your lungs.

# ABOUT THE AUTHOR

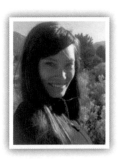 **Julie  Schoen** is an author, yoga instructor, former model, teacher, and co-founder of the company Little Pearl Publishing, dedicated to bringing the world "little pearls" of wisdom.

Over the past six years, Julie Schoen has dedicated her life to pursuing knowledge and sharing it through her writing and teaching. In 2005, she was in a hit-and-run car accident, leaving her with serious injuries to her head and spine. After consulting numerous physical therapists and chiropractors, Schoen turned to yoga and meditation to heal her body and spirit. During the long healing process from this accident, she developed a new gratefulness for life's opportunities and takes advantage of each one that she is given.

As an experienced teacher and yoga instructor, Schoen has traveled the world studying with and absorbing the wisdom of each person she meets. A devoted wife and mom, she is thankful for the opportunity to make a living writing, teaching, and traveling, while still being present for every moment of her life.

**For More Great Books By Julie Check Out**
www.amazon.com/author/julieschoen

**Discover More Brilliant Must-Read Books**
www.amazon.com/author/littlepearl

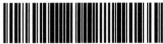

Made in the USA
San Bernardino, CA
31 May 2013